I0415580

How To Prevent Hair Loss

"Hair Fall Treatment For Women And Men"

"Are You Ready To Discover Natural Hair Loss Treatments For Women Or For Men? You Can Use These Hairloss Treatments To Prevent Hair Loss, Or To Regrow Some Hair."

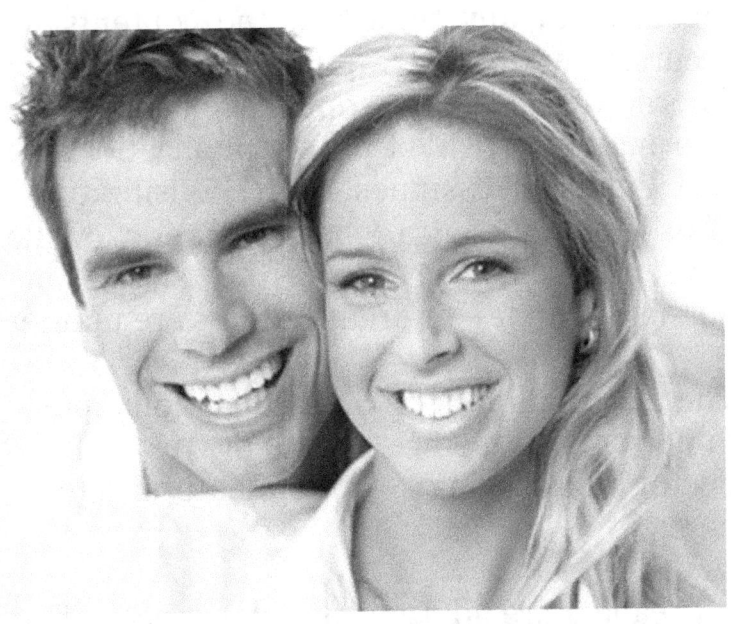

By Rudy S Silva, Natural Nutritionist

How To Prevent Hair Loss © 2013 by Rudy S Silva

ISBN-13: 978-1492959274
ISBN-10: 1492959278

All Rights Reserved. No part of this publication may be reproduced in any form or by any means, including scanning, photocopying, or otherwise without prior written permission of the copyright holder.

Disclaimer and Terms of Use: The Author and Publisher has strived to be as accurate and complete as possible in the creation of this book, notwithstanding the fact that he does not warrant or represent at any time that the contents within are accurate due to the rapidly changing nature of the Internet. While all attempts have been made to verify information provided in this publication, the Author and Publisher assumes no responsibility for errors, omissions, or contrary interpretation of the subject matter herein. Any perceived slights of specific persons, peoples, or organizations are unintentional.

The information here is for educational purposes and in no way is it medical advice or treatment. Ask your doctor before using any of the natural remedies listed here.

All readers are advised to seek services of competent professionals in legal, business, accounting, medical and finance field. Printed in the United States of America

Table of Contents

Introduction What To Expect From This e-Book

To Stop hair loss and grow hair, you need to work on your whole body. You need to rebuild your organs so that they are healthy and work right. There is no magic pill to take or topical cream that will help you recover your hair. So read on and find out what you need to do. This e-book gives you a lot of nutritional information that you can use to prevent, stop, or regrow some hair.

First, I'm not going to lie to you and say that you can actually stop your hair loss or grow the hair that you want. It is difficult to do both, and I am sure that if you have these concerns, you have tried many things to achieve them. But, I will tell you that if you do nothing about this, you will lose a lot of hair and will end up with an unhealthy body.

However, if you are persistent in applying many of the hair health techniques discussed here, you may be able to stop your hair loss, recover some of the hair loss, and for sure improve your health.

There is a lot of mis-information about hair loss throughout the Internet and in written books. First of all, I have read a lot of articles that claim you cannot recover or regrow hair once you lose it and the only way to regain it is by using of drugs. Of course, these articles are written by people selling those drugs.

But, if you read carefully, you can see that re-growing or stopping hair loss is really about getting your body back into nutritional balance and getting your organs back into the best health possible. So if you move in this direction and take this approach, you will preserve the hair you have and perhaps grow a little, and at the same time you will improve your health and live a much longer life.

What I will show you in this book is natural processes and nutritional methods that you can use for caring and feeding your hair.

Everyone experiences hair loss. Men have this issue more than women. But, both suffer from the loss of their hair, and it's a battle for both to maintain their hair beauty.

So, now you can learn some of the secrets that many people and health practitioners keep to themselves. Most people think that hair loss is completely hereditary. Your genes are programmed with instructions for hair growth as provided by your parents and their parents. And, if you live, eat, and think like your parents, then you will have the same type of hair or hair loss they have or had.

Geriatrists say that many genes have tags on them. These tags are chemicals attached to the genes, which modify the genetic instructions. Some of these tags you are born with and some of them you acquire by your diet, the air you breathe, the stress you're exposed to, way you think, and your lifestyle.

Many people ask me if heredity can be overcome when their parents had hair loss. Here is something to consider. By the time you are losing your hair, you have aged to a certain point that certain body functions and organs have deteriorated. Now, it may not be possible to rejuvenate these organs through nutritional supplementation or natural diets. But, if your body's response to nutritional techniques described here, you will see some hair growth and will be able to stop your hair from continuing to thin.

And if you change your diet, eating habits, stress, and lifestyle, you can change the tags attached to specific genes and cause them to move on to another gene or to move elsewhere.

The older you are the slower your hair grows.

But, for those of you that have plenty of hair and it's still thick, then this is the time for you to start using a nutritional plan. A plan that will help you maintain thick and healthy hair. For those of you that still have some hair left, then you too must practice health hair techniques, if you want to keep what you have.

Areas that Affect Hair Loss and Hair Growth

In this book, you will find a variety of methods that

you can use to help minimize hair loss and also to re-grow some of your hair back. How successful you are in doing this will depend on the reasons for your hair loss and how motivated you are to stay on a specific program that you find might help you.

So, I will not waste your time, and I will get straight into the matter you are interested in – how to stop hair loss and start growing hair.

There are 12 areas that you need to consider and concentrate on for hair care. This will give you a chance to stop hair loss or re-grow some of it. Each chapter covers one of these areas.

There is no guarantee that these methods will work for you. For some of you, they will work wonders and for others, they may have no effect. The reason for this is everyone has different genetic coding, emotional stabilities, stressors, nutritional requirement, digestive abilities, and body health conditions.

The combination of these conditions is enormous, and all contribute to how you process and use the various nutritional supplements, diet changes, reduction in stress and improvements in health.

The last-place nutritional supplements go to is your hair. If your hair is lacking silicon and becomes weak and thins out, adding silicon to your diet may not help your hair. The silicon may be needed by other parts of your body, so your body will take it and use it there.

If your hair and thyroid need zinc to be healthy and strong and you eat rich zinc food, your body will send zinc to your thyroid instead of to your hair. A good working thyroid is more important than nice thick shiny hair. It's the way your body prolongs your life.

So simply by doing what I will be showing you for your hair, your body may use it in other areas where it is needed. But, as you stay with a good nutritional plan, your health will get better, and your hair health will improve.

So let get started.

1: What Causes Hair Loss?

Knowing the various causes of hair loss may help you identify why you have hair loss. This will gives you a chance to change these habits or conditions, so you can stop doing some of the things that cause hair loss. Everyone has different reasons why they lose hair or have difficulty growing hair. In the list that follows, you can see why hair loss is a complex health problem. Just as poor skin appearance is a health problem so is hair loss.

Here is a list of the different issues that you need to consider and ask if these conditions exist for you. If they do, I will provide information on ways to improve these conditions or areas. Every little bit that you do will go to assist you to minimize your hair loss. Don't expect results right away. Just choose a program that you can stick to, for many months. Vary your program as you go.

In addition to genetics, various health problems and diseases, such as iron deficiency, diabetes, stress, poor circulation, acute illnesses, vitamin deficiencies, chemotherapy, thyroid disease, poor diet, dieting, and skin diseases, also promote hair loss. In women, hair thinning or hair loss can occur during menopause or childbirth. Or, it can be caused by an imbalance in estrogen and progesterone.

Heart disease

Most of you, over time, develop plaque buildup along your artery walls. This plaque narrows your arteries and reduces the blood circulation throughout your body and scalp. This is a major cause that prevents you from having healthy hair. When plaque builds up along your artery walls, this prevents Nitric Oxide, which is produced by the artery walls, from getting into the blood stream where it can reach the hair follicles to stimulate hair growth.

The less blood that reaches your hair follicles the fewer nutrients and nitric oxide are available for growing hair.

Heredity

Our bodies always work toward what we inherit. Heredity is a strong force. If your parents had or have thinning hair and specific baldness, then this is what you can expect for yourself. This is true if you eat the same diet and live the same life style your parents did. And, general this is what happens, since you lived with them for the first 20 or so years. And, after you're on your own, you continue the eating habits and lifestyle you learned from your parents or created yourself.

Overcoming genetic habits or characteristics are difficult because they are imprinted in your DNA, genes, and cells and represent a strong force. So you need a stronger force to change these imprinted genetics. This is done by providing a strong dose of the vitamins or minerals that are lacking. Minerals have magnetic and electrical charges that are passed on to cells during metabolism. This is why the right type and amount of a lacking mineral can change various conditions that relate to genetics.

Minerals build cells, tissue, bones, hair, and muscles.

The original intention of your genetics may have been to have a full set of hair. But, since there may have been a lack of hair nutrients in your childhood diet, this could have set the stage for your hair loss as an adult.

But knowing this, you can make changes in your life style. You can learn to eat healthier, take the supplements your hair needs, care for your cardiovascular system, and exercise more. This will result in interfering with heredity for the better. But the sooner you interrupt a poor lifestyle, the better chance you have of having a good head of hair, for a long time.

Drugs

Use of drugs also causes hair loss. This occurs because drugs deplete your body's minerals by passing them out your urine or stools. If you use anti-fungal or a bronchodilators, you will lose the mineral potassium. If you use anti-diabetic drugs, you will lose iodine. If you use anti-thyroid, aspirin, diuretics, or tetracyclines, you will lose calcium, phosphorus, magnesium, and zinc.

Drugs upset the mineral balance in your body. This imbalance leads to disease. It's an undesirable cycle where the long term use of drugs leads to the depletion of the very minerals you need to bring about a recovery.

Dieting and Weight Loss

Being on a diet to lose weight can cause you to lose hair. When you are on a diet, your goal is to lose weight and not to improve your health. Eating less food and less nutritional food reduces your mineral intake. This affects the function of your enzyme activity, digestive and elimination system, pancreas, liver, thyroid, and adrenals. Your body becomes unbalanced in the nutrients it needs to keep your body and hair healthy.

If you change your diet to vegetarian, then you run the risk of losing hair, if you don't eat enough protein.

Women and Hair Loss

Women lose their hair differently than men. Women lose hair throughout their scalp, and their hair thins out, whereas men become bald in certain spots base on heredity. A woman's hormones and heredity determine the growth cycle of their hair and, as they age, the growth cycle shortens. The result is their hair does not grow as long and thick as before.

However, just as with men, DHT has an influence on women's follicle roots, and an excess of DHT will undermine them.

Women tend to see hair loss during changes in their hormones, which occur during child birth or menopause.

During menopause, women experience a decrease in estrogen, and this causes an increase in testosterone. This increase in testosterone can be converted to DHT.

Women, prior to 1950, had little hair loss or thinning. After 1955, women's hair loss increased and now one in three women experiences hair loss. This change is women's hair health appears to be associated with the emergence of new shampoos with new chemical additives, new chemical hair preparations, use of more pharmaceuticals, poor nutritional habits, use of tight hair preparations and styles – pony tails, teasing, permanent wave, rollers- and stress.

Always look for those products that are natural and have fewer petrochemical additives – it's those chemicals in ingredients that are hard to pronounce – propylene glycol, lauramide DEA, sodium laureth, ammonium lauryl sulfate,

Other bad additives are:

quaternium-22, acrylates, dimethylamine lactate, dyes, distearate quaternary -26, squalane, TEAcarbonmer 934, benzyl alcohol

And there are hundreds more un-natural chemicals that are added to shampoos, hair gels, or hair conditioners.

One other thing, women need to be careful about it is dyeing their hair. Dyeing their hair can cause hair to thin and become brittle. If you really need to dye it, look for natural dyeing products that will not harm your hair.

Out of Balanced Hormones lead to Hair Loss

The hormones – testosterone, estrogen, and DHT - and nutrients flowing in your blood determine the health of your hair. To change your blood chemistry takes around 3 month provided you're feeding yourself the right nutrients. It is the improved blood nutrients that will rebuild your body organs and systems.

Using natural hair topical treatments can be used to enhance the nutrients that you have in your blood.

Trapped Blood Plasma Protein

One of the secrets to having good health and growing hair is to reduce the amount of blood plasma protein that leaks out of your blood vessels and ends up hiding and accumulating around your cell structures. Normally blood plasma protein is supposed to stay in your arteries, veins, and capillaries. Its molecules are too large to pass through these blood vessel walls, unless you have an injury, eat toxic chemicals, are poisoned, have stress, then these vessel wall pores enlarge and the blood plasma protein seeps out into the lymph liquid.

So why is blood plasma protein in your lymph bad for you? Because this protein attracts water and becomes bonded with the sodium in the lymph. This causes water to accumulate around the cells, preventing them from receiving its share of nutrients and excreting its metabolized waste. This excess water prevents the cell from get enough oxygen causing the cell to become sick and diseased. In your scalp, your cells become weak and unable to support hair growth

Hair Mites

There is a tiny mite that lives in practically all hair follicles called Demodex follicularum. This mite can be a cause or can contribute to your hair loss. It is thought that the difference between people who lose hair and those who don't is in how the scalp reacts to these mites.

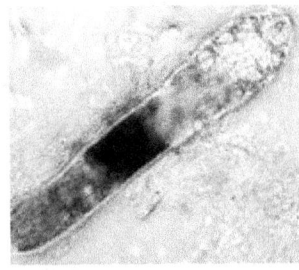 If your body has an inflammatory reaction to these mites in an effort to eliminate them, the follicle may close down killing the mite but also killing the hair. (Photo from: Microscopy UK or

their contributors) The Demodex mite is frequently found around face follicles or deep into the sebaceous gland that releases sebum oil. This mite is considered a parasite, which usually does not bother us except as we get older. Perhaps it's because as we get older, our immune system gets weaker.

This mite exists in larger quantities when you have an oily face or hair, since they feed on the sebum secreted by the sebaceous gland. In large quantities, these mites, which are parasites, are known to cause abnormal hair loss. Their feeding on sebum robs the hair of its nutrients, causing the hair to fall out. These mites are not found on everyone. They are found in 90% of the men or women that have thinning hair.

Life Style and Hair Loss

Lifestyle determines the chemistry in your blood and this in turn determines the health of your hair. If you are losing your hair, look at your lifestyle and decide if you have to change it.

Unfortunately, most of us worry about hair loss when we see we are losing hair. When this happens, hair loss, most likely, is a result of unhealthy eating and lifestyle patterns. Of course, when you see you are losing hair, you may resolve to do something about it, but then you might find it is difficult to do. Not only is it difficult to do, it is hard to get good information on what you can do for your hair loss.

In his book, The Magic of Herbs in Daily Living, 1972, Richard Lucas writes about, "Another case involved that of a man Pat middle age with a history of weak glands, which was completely bald on top except for a few long hairs.

He had tried ointments, heat lamps, massage and other things. Nothing worked.

When he heard the diet theory, he began giving up some of the foods he had formerly eaten and substituting those recommended. He started out by eating sunflower seeds, about one cup for breakfast. Then he tried sunflower seed meal along with pumpkin seed meal and other natural foods. In a few months he noticed a few black hairs at the temple, and then he started in earnest to see what he could do about growth.

After another 18 months a progress report on this case showed that the subject was doing so well in growing hair that he was able to reduce some of his supplements. He no longer needed to take the B-complex tablets and this dose of vegetable and wheat germ oil were reduced to about one teaspoonful a day. He also cut down on the amount of meat in his diet.

Apparently, some younger men have accomplished in weeks what this older man with his sluggish glands, and many health problems did in years."

What this case shows is it is possible to grow hair

even if you are bald in certain areas. The question really is are you willing to put in the effort to get your organs back to health, so they can do what is necessary to give you a healthy body and a head full of hair.

2: How Your Hair Grows

I am sure many of you have read about how hair grows in cycles. However, I will repeat this information because I will be referring back to it, and it will help you to have this information in your mind as you read this e-book.

Your scalp has around 125,000 follicles and about 500,000 glands that provide water, oil, and nourishment to your follicles, hair, and scalp. Keeping these glands healthy is necessary for strong and lasting hair.

The follicle, a hollow shaft, is where your hair shaft resides. At the base of the follicle is the papilla, where your hair root resides. This is where protein is created and provides carbon, hydrogen, nitrogen, sulfur, and oxygen to create keratin. These are the ingredients necessary to make your hair cells.

The sebaceous gland, which is located along side of the hollow follicle, provides a yellowish lubricant called sebum. Sebum oil keeps your hair from becoming brittle and splitting. With it moisture content, sebum keeps surrounding tissue moist and keeps your scalp from drying. Depending on how much sebum oil is released from your follicles, this will determine if you have dry or oily scalp. One problem with sebum is when you excrete excess amounts, it promotes hair loss.

Your scalp, normally, will scale off skin and this scale will lie on your scalp or hair. Excess scaling is known as dandruff and in severe cases, it is called seborrhea.

To keep the sebaceous and sebum healthy, you need to eat foods with plenty of omega-3, omega-6, and omega-9 oils. You can also get the essential omega oils by supplementing with fish or flax seed oil. You need to take minerals to keep your sebum healthy.

The Hair Growing Cycles

Your hair grows in three cycles, anlagen, cartage, and deluge. The anlagen cycle is the growing period. Your hair is in this cycle 85% of the time and lasts for about 2 – 6 years. Your hair is capable of growing two inches each month.

In the cartage cycle, your hair is in a transitional phase, moving from the anlagen to the deluge cycle.

In the deluge cycle, your hair growth is in a resting period. It is in this cycle for about 3 months. When your hair starts to regrow, this new hair will push out the old hair causing it to fall.

When your new hair emerges onto your scalp, it is essentially dead tissue. It is not capable of repair or regeneration and is subject to abuse from detrimental shampoo chemicals and other hair products. It is also subjected to physical abuse from hair brushes, special hairdos, or hair dryers.

The only living part of your hair is the hair root, bulb shaped, which is located at the bottom of the follicle shaft. It is filled with capillaries that bring in the nutrients that you have eaten. The hair root is only capable of supplying two hairs. Once you have lost one, you have just one left during your life. Two nutrients that your hair root requires are iodine and iron.

When you have a full head of hair, you lose as many hairs as you grow hairs. For many years, you see only thick hair. In time, you start to lose more hair than is replaced.

So, why do more hairs fallout than are replaced? The following sections will answer this question. It is usually more than one thing that causes excess hair loss. It is a combination of health issues, and this is the reason it is so hard to regrow or to stop hair loss.

The hair shaft consists of three layers, the medulla, the cortex, and the cuticle. The medulla is the inner middle layer or the core of your hair, and if you have thin hair, it does not exist. It is the supporting structure of your hair and is capable of absorbing beneficial substances that are rubbed onto your hair.

The cortex is the layer surrounding the medulla and is the second inner layer. It is this layer that provides your hair strength and flexibility. It also provides your hair with the pigmentation that determines your hair color.

The cuticle is the outmost layer of your hair and is composed of overlapping cells and is capable of absorbing moisture or other chemically that you put on your hair. When you damage your hair, it is this layer that becomes affected. The condition and health of the cuticle determines the appearance of your hair.

The cuticle provides your hair with elasticity and resiliency.

Hair grows faster in the summer and slower in the winter. In those locations where it is warm all the time, hair grows faster than in cold locations. Hair grows faster when it experiences heat and friction as in massage. In those areas where the temperature is always cold hair growth slows down.

3: How to Improve Your Scalp Circulation

Blood circulation through your scalp provides the nutrients to the papilla and hair root that you need for healthy hair and normal growth. Anything that hampers this circulation will affect your hair health and will lead to hair loss and baldness. Here are some conditions that could exist:

Narrowing of the arteries to the head decreases blood circulation to the scalp. This brings less blood to your scalp and fewer hair nutrients to your hair.

Your blood has good circulation to your head, but does not have the right nutrients for good hair growth.

The galena, the crown scalp, thickens and becomes tense, as you age, and reduce the blood circulation to that area.

When you start to experience hair loss, this is a signal that your health is not in balance. It is a good time to take notice and do something about your health. Researchers have found that when you start to develop hardening of the arteries – a condition where atherosclerotic plaque accumulates along artery walls - less nitric oxide (NO) is excreted from the artery walls.

Nitric oxide is needed to keep new hair growing, which replaces old hair that falls out. It is Nitric oxide that is the active ingredient in the product Rogaine. Men who are found with less artery plaque buildup have shown to have more hair than men with excess plaque buildup. Unfortunately, what this means is that men who lose their hair early have an issue with hardening of the arteries and most likely will die of a heart attack or a cardiovascular disease as they age.

Women seem to overcome this problem of reduced nitric release because of their higher estrogen levels

So what must you do to improve nitric oxide release? You must use those supplements and natural remedies that can reverse the plaque buildup along your artery walls.

Scalp stimulators

Here's how you can get more blood to circulate through your scalp and bring more nutrients to your hair follicles. After you shower, if you have a shower hose extension, shower with hot water on your head, as hot as you can stand it, for 15 seconds or so. Then turn the hot water off and let the cold water run over your head for 15 seconds. Do this 4 to 6 times every time you shower. This should take about an extra 5 minutes in the shower. This hot and cold-water application will also keep your ears and brain active and sharp.

When you finish, your will feel refreshed and awake. You may not need coffee and may even decide to eat fruits for breakfast. It is fruit that contains minerals for your hair.

Lack of minerals chromium and manganese with excess fat and sugar in your diet can contribute to the narrowing of arteries leading to the scalp. Available chromium and manganese can help the body digest fats before the can settle on artery walls.

4: How To Deal With DHT Effects

This section is for men, since it deals with the health of the prostate, but women should also be concerned about DHT, since their hair loss can be related to DHT.

The prostate is the considered a sex organ, since it effects man's sexual performance, if it is enlarged, cancerous, or removed during surgery. It is in the prostate where excess testosterone is changed to DHT, di-hydro-testosterone, through a chemical reaction with the enzyme 5 alpha (a) – reductase.

Now, when testosterone is changed to DHT by the 5 alpha (a) – reductase, DHT is called bad testosterone, since it causes the prostate to enlarge and malfunction. The other thing that occurs is some of the DHT is not used up in the prostate, enters the blood stream and ends up at the root of your hair. Here, it interferes with the growth and health of your hair. The result is your hair starts to thin and disappear.

There are various nutrients and supplements that reduce or inhibit the ability of the 5 alpha reductase enzyme to convert testosterone to DHT and this will help you maintain long hair longer.

Here are the nutrients that help to block or reduce the conversion of testosterone to DHT, the bad testosterone.

Pumpkin seed oil – 1000mg per day – provides minerals and zinc.

- Saw palmetto berries extract improves prostate health
- Nettle root extract – improves prostate health
- Bee pollen –improves prostate health
- Borage oil, 1000 mg per day
- Evening primrose oil, 1000 mg, 2-4 time per day
- Fish oil
- Zinc 20 -30 mg per day
- Normal cholesterol levels – reduces formation of DHT
- Beta sitosterol supplement

Beta Sitosterol Products

Here is a product that contains a high level of beta sitosterol. It is used to reduce the amount of testosterone that is converted to DHT. Remember that DHT will make you lose your hair and cause prostate enlargement. Having an enlarged prostate causes excess urination, especially at night. Typically, you may find that you need to get up 2-5 times a night to urinate. Check out Prostate Power Rx, with **beta-sitosterol** to gain control of excessive urinating and DHT.

Stop Hair Loss from Plugged up Hair Follicles

So many men and women start losing their hair when their hair follicles start plugging. Follicle plugging starts early, when you have plenty of hair. And this is the time you should be concerned about how to stop hair loss. Most people worry about hair loss after they start seeing a lot of hair loss. Unfortunately, there are few practitioners writing articles about "stop hair loss," for people that have a full head of hair.

Hair follicles get plugged from within the follicle and from contaminates outside the follicle. Testosterone is a major element in hair loss. When excess testosterone is converted to DHT by the enzyme 5 alpha reductase, DHT interferes with your hair growth by preventing your hair roots from absorbing nutrients. In addition it causes excess sebum to accumulate in the follicle shaft and sets the stage for follicle plugging.

5: Use Natural Products on Your Hair

How to Clean up Your Scalp

Hair Washing — washing your hair with hair shampoos or rinses that contain many unknown chemicals or petroleum derivatives have a damaging effect on your hair. The strength of your hair is affected, and the chemicals tend to pull up your hair follicle.

When you use un-natural shampoos, hair conditioners, gels, and other hair products, these products leave chemical residues on your scalp. These residues combine with dirt, dandruff, dead skin, and oil to form a slime that slips into the follicle and causes follicle plugging.

If you continue to use un-natural hair products, the slime that is created on your scalp will eventually start to harden, plugging up your hair follicles. With plugged follicles, your scalp becomes smooth where hair is buried, and you become bald.

Not only do un-natural shampoos cause hair loss, they also affect your health. The chemicals found in these shampoos, such as propylene glycol, glycol, cetearyl alcohol, methylparaben, propylparaben, distearate, or isopropyl alcohol, can enter your blood stream through your scalp causing damage to your body tissue and cells.

It is always best to use natural hair products, which support and nourish your hair. Look for hair products that have no un-natural additives. I have been making my own shampoos in which I add herbs that are beneficial to hair and scalp.

So what does it all boil down to? Your hair is a measure of your health. The more hair you have, the healthier you are. You can see that as you age you slowly lose your hair and health. This does not need to happen.

When you have a full head of hair, you don't even think about it. And for sure, you don't worry about losing it. But, this is the time to think about your hair and your health. Start learning what it takes to be healthy, take action and your hair will thrive.

Discover what nutrient your body needs to control hair loss and start eating the foods that provide this. You cannot get good nutrients from fast-food restaurants and from frying your food all the time. You cannot get good nutrients from eating canned and package foods. And, you cannot rely on restaurants to feed you nutritious food. This is something you need to decide for yourself. Do you want to keep your hair, stop hair loss, or do you want to lose your hair for good.

When out in the sun, wear a hat or scarf to protect your hair from the damaging effects of UV light. Avoid the use of blow drying, hot curlers, curling irons on your hair. Just pat dry your hair with a towel.

After swimming in a pool or sea, wash your hair to eliminate chlorine. Rotate your shampoo and conditioner every two weeks or so to avoid build-up of the detergents of that shampoo. Look for natural shampoos that don't have petrochemical products.

Types of shampoo to use to prevent hair loss

Use only natural shampoos that will not harm or stress your hair, scalp, and body. Look at the label and buy those shampoos that restore your scalp to a normal pH.

Start using shampoos and conditioners that have silica, biotin, vitamin C and E, Aloe vera gel and jojoba oils. You can use a small squirt of 100% jojoba oil on your hair after you shower and dry your hair. Jojoba oil helps to keep your hair follicles clean and free of dirt and contamination buildup.

Natural herbal shampoo

Here is a natural shampoo that you can make yourself. Buy the following soap and herbs. These items can be purchased at most nutritional stores or health-food stores. If you can't find them there, head to the Internet.

- 8 oz of Castile soap with any scent is that available – plain, peppermint, eucalyptus – peppermint is a good choice

- ½ oz of rosemary - stimulates the hair follicles and helps to prevent premature baldness

- ½ oz of sage – has antioxidants and keeps things from spoiling and is antibacterial

- ½ oz of nettles – acts as a blood purifier, blood stimulator, contains a large source of nutrients for hair growth

- ½ of lavender – controls the production of sebaceous gland oil and reduces itchy and flaky scalp conditions

- 2000 mg of MSM – provides organic sulfur to your scalp, which improves the health and strength of your hair. It also helps to drive herbal nutrients into the skin and follicles where they can do the most good

- One empty 8 oz. plastic bottle or any other empty shampoo or soap bottle

Mix the herbs in a mason jar, which has a lid. Shake and twist the jar to mix the herbs. Boil 1 1/2 cups of distilled water. Add 3 heaping tablespoons of the mixed herbs into the boiling water. Let the herbs boil over low heat for 5 minutes. Pull the boiling water and herbs off the stove.

Let the herb mixture sit for 25 – 30 minutes, then strain the herbal mixture into a bowl or cup with a sprout. After 30 minutes, put 2000mg of MSM into the herb mixture.

Pour 4 oz. of strained herbal infusion into an 8 oz plastic bottle. Now, pour the 3 1/2 oz. of Castile soap into the 8 oz. plastic bottle. Finally, add 1 to 2 tablespoons of apple cider vinegar to for pH balance and as a preservative. Cap the bottle and shake to mix the ingredients.

The shampoo is now finished and ready for use. Use this as a base for all the shampoos you make. You can add different herbs as you learn what these herbs do and how they help your hair. You can vary the ingredients according to your taste. But now you have a shampoo that has no additives that can't harm you.

Egg shampoo

This shampoo is only good for three days or so, and you have to store it in the refrigerator after each use. Use this shampoo for the three days then use the other herbal shampoo for the other four days. The egg shampoo is designed to provide your hair and follicles with protein or amino acids that your hair and hair follicles need to keep strong, healthy, and promote hair growth. The fresh egg in this shampoo provides this needed protein. Using regular eggs is ok but I use organic or free range eggs.

Put the following ingredients into a blender:

Break one egg into a blender A teaspoon or less of 98% aloe
Vera gel

Three or four squirts of Jojoba oil and 2000 mg of MSM. If you use powdered MSM capsules, break them open and drop the powder into the blender but not the capsules. If you use MSM torpedoes, just drop them into the blender. The MSM helps to deliver the blended egg protein into your hair and scalp.

Add three tablespoons of apple cider vinegar

Add quarter cup or less of Castile liquid soap

Turn on the blender to blend this mixture. After about 1-2 minutes of blending, check to see what consistency you have. You want this mixture to flow thickly into your plastic bottle. If it is too thick to flow add a little more Castile soap or a tablespoon of water and blend a little longer. You can experiment a little with this formula to get it to flow easily.

Now, pour it into an 8 or 16 oz. plastic bottle. The egg shampoo is now ready to feed your scalp. You can wash your hair with it in a sink and then let the shampoo stay on your hair for 5 – 10 minutes, or you can shower and wash your hair many times and let it stay on your hair for 5 minutes or so.

Apple Cider or Lemon Hair Rinse

Your hair and scalp are normally slightly acidic, a pH of 4.5 to 5.5, which helps to control and kill germs that would otherwise accumulate. This pH is also necessary for your scalp cells to completely metabolize protein into amino acids, which your cells and follicles use as food. When your scalp cells are able to use these amino acids, they have the best elasticity, strength, and shine. You will be providing this protein in the egg shampoo.

Maintaining the proper scalp pH is necessary for you to have healthy hair. Most commercial shampoos leave your hair pH alkaline, from 7.0 and up. This weakens your hair and promotes hair loss. Some shampoos are labeled pH balance, which mean they leave your scalp pH 4.5 to 5.5.

Here's how you can make your scalp pH balanced. You can use apple cider vinegar or lemon juice.

Prepare an apple cider hair-rinse or lemon-rinse to be used before or after you shampoo your hair. Here's how to make it.

In an 8 oz plastic bottle pour 4 - 6 oz of apple cider vinegar or squeeze the juice of one or two lemon. Then, add distilled or reverse osmosis water to fill the rest of the bottle. The apple cider or lemon hair rinse is now ready for use.

Using the Apple Cider Rinse

Just before you wash your hair, put the apple cider rinse into your hair to change the pH of your scalp. This is necessary to get the best benefits of the egg shampoo.

Sometimes after I use the herbal shampoo, I do a final rinse using the apple cider rinse, and I do this while I am in the shower.

Aloe Vera Gel and Jojoba Oil

After your hair is dry you can mix in your hand some aloe vera gel and jojoba oil and run it into your scalp and hair. You can experiment on the mixture and amount you need for your hair.

Dry Hair

One important supplement to take for dry hair is the essential fatty acids. Use them daily in the form of flax seed oil, borage oil, or fish oil. Look at the labels of the foods you eat to avoid those oils that have been partial hydrogenated or hydrogenated. Using oils that are hydrogenated, keep your immune system weak. These hydrogenated oils are stored as toxins in your body. Then, when you detoxify your body, it will be release acidic waste.

Hair Brush

When you use the right kind of hair brush and keep it clean you will have strong, healthy, hair, which will not fall out in the future. Then by taking a Collagen and Hyaluronic Acid supplement, you can strengthen your hair.

Hair care starts when you brush your hair. There are at least three things you need to know about how to brush your hair to bring more blood circulation to your scalp. Increasing the blood circulation to your scalp keeps your hair strong.

A Natural Hair Brush

Use a natural bristle like boar's hair. Boar bristles are similar to the keratin of your hair and absorb the dirt and oil just like your hair. In addition, the tips of the boar hair brush are rounded and gently massage your scalp and hair.

Kent hair brushes are available in boar hair. But, avoid the Kent nylon hair brush, if you want the best care for your hair.

The nylon hair brush is not recommended, since it is rougher on your scalp and is nowhere as good as the boar bristle hair brush. The nylon bristles are usually sharp and inflamed your follicles and break your hair.

Brushing Your Hair

To maintain excellent hair growth you need good circulation to your scalp. You also need a clean scalp, with little oil and dirt accumulating in your hair follicles. The boar hair brush helps you achieve this, when you regularly brush your hair.

Brush your hair when it is dry. This prevents your hair from breaking. When you brush, the gentle pulling of your hair stimulates your scalp bringing in more blood to feed your hair. Also, the slight pulling stimulates the release of oil from your follicles, which lubricates your hair.

Brush your hair with a boar bristle hair brush twice a day for the best hair care – morning and night. For short hair, brush for three minutes and for long hair brush five minutes.

By bending your head to the floor, when brushing, you will increase the blood circulation to your scalp. Now, brush from your neck forward to the front of your scalp, then, from sides to your crown. Lastly, brush your hair from the front of your scalp to the neck.

Cleaning Your Boar Hair Brush

If possible, you should clean your brush every day. If you have two or more hair brushes, then it will be easier to do this. Your boar bristle hair brush will accumulate dirt and oils from your hair when you brush. Without regular cleaning of your hair brush, this dirt and oil will redeposit onto your hair. Over time this added dirt and oil will plug up your hair follicles and lead to hair thinning or permanent hair loss.

You can clean your brush every day, when you shower. You can clean it with shampoo and scrub the bristles with your hand back and forth. After cleaning, you can dry the brush with a towel and let it sit until the next day. By the next day, it is ready to use it and your second brush is set to be cleaned.

So, using a natural hair brush like the boar bristle hair brush is the best way to care for your hair. Gentle daily brushing stimulates your scalp and keeps your hair healthy.

6: Improve Your Thyroid Function

Having Thyroid Hormone Deficiencies of Thyroxin (T4), And Triiodothyronine (T3), will cause hair loss and poor health.

To have good hair growth your thyroid has to produce the amount of thyroxine your body needs. One of the first things to do, in your hair growth program, is to check your thyroid output.

Recently Will Brink, health researcher and writer, wrote an article about how excess thyroid-stimulating hormone, TSH, which is released by the pituitary gland, can cause low thyroid function, or hypothyroidism. This happens when your thyroid is weak and needs extra thyroid-stimulating hormone to get it working properly.

But, sometimes when the thyroid is putting out low amount of hormones, no amount of extra thyroid-stimulating hormone from the pituitary gland will stimulate the thyroid to put out more thyroxine hormone.

If this is the case with your thyroid, chances are that your thyroid is working below average in releasing it own hormone, thyroxine. And, when you are under a lot of stress, your thyroxine may be used up on its way to your cells.

Thyroid Suppressors

Chemicals

Your thyroid function is also suppressed by heavy metals such as mercury, cadmium, and lead. It is suppressed by fluoride in the water and in toothpaste. I recommend using natural or non-fluorinated toothpastes. Cigarette smoke also suppresses the thyroid function.

Getting radiation exposure is the worst thing you can do to your thyroid. For this reason, you should always insist on lead protect for your thyroid, when getting dental or other x-rays.

Diet

One of the most harmful foods that affect your thyroid is those that have genetically engineered or have synthetic hormones – meat, poultry, eggs, and dairy products.

Iodine, which is needed for good thyroid function, can have the reverse effect, if you consume too much of it. Iodine is found in dough conditioner, salt, and kelp.

Vegetables like cabbage, broccoli or cauliflower have thyroid suppressing chemicals, which can be deactivated by slightly steaming them. Soy has been found to be detrimental for the thyroid and excess use of safflower and corn oils also have the same effect.

Deficiencies in vitamin A, B, copper, iron, selenium and zinc also slow down the thyroid.

If you know you have low thyroid output – hypothyroidism, limit your use of peanuts, soy, flour, millet, walnuts and apples. The vegetables you should avoid are cabbage, spinach, mustard greens, kale, Brussels sprouts, cauliflower, turnips, and broccoli.

Stress

Adrenaline and cortical, which are released when you have stress, interferes with the conversion of the thyroid hormone T4 to T3. T3 is the more active thyroid hormone which runs your body. As less T4 is converted to T3, the more adrenaline and cortisol are released and a vicious cycle sets up.

Thyroid triiodothyronine and thyroxine hormones are needed by every body cell to help convert nutrients into the body energy you need. Without this energy, your whole body slows down, including your brain, and you feel run down, depressed, and find it difficult to concentrate.

When you have a weak thyroid and low thyroxine output, you may have symptoms that you may not associate with your thyroid. In fact, these symptoms can be related to other health problems.

Here is some of the symptoms associated hypothyroidism, low thyroxine output.

- You feel fatigued, tired or run down
- You have trouble concentrating
- You have depression and bad moods
- You're cranky and difficult to get along with
- You have irregular periods and may have difficulty
- getting pregnant
- You feel cold when other people feel warm
- Your hair starts to fall out or thin down
- You may develop constipation
- You may have increase cholesterol levels
- You start to gain weight
- You may develop hoarseness in your voice
- You develop a slow heart beat

Many of us have low levels of thyroxine and we don't know. I know that in the past, I have tested myself and discovered that I had hypothyroidism. Now recent research has associated hypothyroidism with the cardiac condition Tachycardia. Tachycardia is a heart condition that causes the heart to beat more than 100 beats per minute.

You can test to see if you have hypothyroidism using the basal method. In this method, you measure your underarm temperature with a basal thermometer four or more days in a row.

Your natural temperature should be between 97.2 F and 98.2 F. If your temperature is down at 97.2 F, you may want to raise it back to normal at 97.7 F or even to 98.0F. Of course, if it is lower or higher than normal, you would want to consult with your doctor.

To measure your body temperature it is best to use a glass thermometer and not a digital one. The thermometer accuracy you need is 0.1 F. Mercury thermometers are no longer made because of toxicity. It is now hard to find have good thermometers.

Diet and Nutrients for good thyroid function

For a healthy thyroid, here is the food you need to concentration on:

Seaweed, dulse, kelp, garlic, watercress, radishes, egg yolks, seafood, fruit juices, watermelon and coconut oil

Aloe vera juice has also been helpful in improving thyroid function. You can take it as a juice. Sometimes when I make a smoothie, I put a tablespoon of the gel into the blender.

Use organic sea salt instead of iodized salt. Coconut oil is the healthiest saturated fat that can stimulate thyroid function.

For low thyroid function, doctors will typically prescribe:

A synthetic thyroid hormone, thyroxine or triiodothyronine

A desiccated pork thyroid gland, which contains certain amounts of thyroid hormone – the main brand is Armour Thyroid.

Now, you can purchase a thyroid tissue extract over the Internet or at your health-food store. This extract is allowed over the counter since, by law, it cannot contain any active thyroid hormones. Most alternative practitioners will recommend this extract, since they feel it will build and support your thyroid.

For my low basal temperature reading, I purchased Pure Encapsulations **Thyroid Support Complex** and was able to bring my body temperature back to normal.

7: Nutritional Supplements that Feed Your Hair

Hair growth occurs at the hair root in the papilla and in the root is living tissue or cells. Blood brings nutrients to the hair root, which it uses to grow hair. What you have in the blood is what determines the nutrients your hair will get. If your hair is thinning, falling out, brittle or split, or turning gray prematurely, then you need to take those minerals and vitamins that feed your hair, for a minimum of 3 months, before you start to see improvement.

When your hair does not receive the nutrients, it needs the papillae, which houses the root of your hair, will contract, wither, and die.

Your hair needs the B vitamins, minerals, and special nutrients. If you are under stress, you will quickly use up your nutrients, and they will not reach your scalp or hair. Your hair is the last place nutrients go to. If your body needs nutrients, your hair will get very little.

The fact that you're short on nutrients will affect your overall health and start you on the path to high blood pressure, arteriosclerosis, heart problems, or other diseases. This path is a downward spiral that continues to impact your hair, resulting in thinning and balding. You are living up to your heredity.

Of course, your nutrition is affected by how your body works. If you have thyroid, digestion, liver, colon, kidney, heart, and other body issues, the amount of nutrients available for your cells and hair will be diminished. Nutrients go to where they are most needed.

Eat plenty of fruits and vegetables and back off on the starches, protein, and fatty foods. Fruits contain flavonoids, which are antioxidants that protect the hair follicles and promote hair growth.

Add flax seeds or flax seed oil to your diet. Flax seed oil helps to reduce inflammation at the hair follicle. In addition, it prevents the build of androgens at the hair follicle. Androgens cause the follicle to become inflamed, and this causes them to shut down or close off.

The food you eat will determine what nutrients are available for your hair root. Eat a fast food diet and your hair gets little or no nutrients, and you will have many other health problems.

Your hair needs a lot of B-vitamins and minerals. You can choose those foods that contain these nutrients. Use vegetables and fruits, since they are high in vitamins and minerals. Use an ionic or liquid mineral supplement.

Here is a list of Minerals and Vitamins that are necessary for good hair health. If your hair is deficient in these nutrients, then you will possibly have hair loss.

- Vitamin A
- Biotin
- Brewer's or nutritional yeast
- Collagen
- Copper
- choline
- Folic Acid
- Inositol
- Iodine
- Lysine
- Oxygen
- estrogen
- Pantothenic Acid
- Phosphorus
- Selenium
- Silicon
- Testosterone
- Vitamin C
- Vitamin E
- Wheat germ
- Zinc

Vitamin A

Vitamin A is required for general body health and is definitely needed for good hair health. By combining

Vitamin A with Silica and Zinc, the sebaceous gland is prevented from drying up or clogging. When the sebaceous gland clogs, your hair can become dry and dull, and you could develop dandruff. Lack of these nutrients, can cause your scalp to thicken and trap oil and moisture underneath it surface. Vitamin A is also needed for good thyroid health. Also, Iodine is needed for thyroid function and to keep the papilla, hair root, healthy.

Vitamin A is destroyed by smoking, air pollution, drugs, and laxatives. This vitamin is fat soluble and is stored in the body. The foods that are high in vitamin A are:

Alfalfa, beets, broccoli, apricots, cantaloupes, carrots, swiss chard, fish liver oil, kale, parsley, red peppers, sweet potatoes, spinach, yellow squash, and watercress.

B-Vitamin Complex

The B-vitamins are one of the most important vitamins to take if you expect to stop hair loss or grow hair. Men need more than women. And, there are a lot of body conditions that destroy these vitamins, such as stress or excess exercising. Eating processed foods will make you deficient in B vitamins, since B vitamins are needed in digesting processed foods.

Since B vitamins are water soluble, they are easily loss from vegetables or grains that are heated, boiled or over cooked. But just taking them alone will not grow your hair.

Biotin – is a B vitamin and has shown signs of slowing down hair loss. Without biotin, your body does not use protein, amino acids, or fats effectively. Biotin produces amino acids that are used in creating hair. So, in addition to other health reasons, you don't want to be short of biotin.

You get biotin in three ways – by your intestines producing it, by eating certain foods, and by taking supplements.

So, for your intestines to produce it, you need to have plenty of good bacteria or what is called probiotics. So, take a good probiotic supplement. There are many on the market, and you should just rotate monthly from one to another.

Here is one to consider **NOW Foods Probiotic-10** Note that stress kills the good bacteria in your intestines leading to less biotin produced. So what are the symptoms when you lack biotin? They are,

- Dry scaly skin
- Anorexia
- Seborrheic dermatitis
- Alopecia (hair loss)
- Nausea

So, for hair loss, you need to make sure any multi-supplement you take has biotin. As a supplement, you should take up to 300 mcg of biotin (micrograms.)

In addition, you need to take a good probiotic supplement.

Here are the foods that have biotin:

Organ meats, eggs, mushrooms, nuts, peanuts, cauliflower, whole wheat, rice bran, walnuts, pecans, oatmeal, lentils brown rice. Salt water fish, soybeans, chicken, and nutritional yeast

Brewer's yeast has the highest contain of biotin of all of these foods. Go to here to get Brewer's Yeast at Amazon.

Inositol – is another B vitamin, which protects hair follicles. It does this by forming lecithin, which in turn reduces the damaging effects of fats and cholesterol on follicle walls and tissue. This helps to prevent hair loss. Inositol is also known to reduce stress, and this helps to increase blood circulation. When you drink coffee the levels of Inositol are reduced.

Inositol foods – tomatoes, eggs, watermelon, cabbage, cauliflower, onions, strawberries, brown rice, raisins, oranges, navy beans, barley, wheat germ, green peas, grapefruit, and cantaloupe.

Oxygen – is the most important substance you need for survival. Oxygen helps you metabolize nutrients in your cells to create the energy you need to run your body. It also is a detoxifier that breaks down toxins for elimination and destroys all sorts of pathogens that harm you or create disease.

By taking oxygen with various supplements and good food that you take to stop hair loss or to grow hair, you will enhance your chances of growing hair.

Oxygen helps you get rid of toxins and thereby improves your immunity. When this happens, your body functions better and can then do some of the functions it was intended to, like grow or stop hair loss.

There are two ways to get more oxygen into your body – improve your breathing and take stabilized O2.

Selenium – is important in keeping the thyroid hormones in balance. Remember you need a thyroid that can put out sufficient hormones to give your body the energy it needs to function. Selenium also acts as an antioxidant and helps to keep heavy metals from accumulating in your hair.

When you read the selenium supplement label, make sure you don't buy or use sodium selenite, since it is not freely absorbed. Use seleno-methionine, which is chelated and passes easily through your intestines.

Keep your dose of selenium to 200-300 mcg per day, unless your doctor asks you to take more. You can overdose on this mineral, but it seldom occurs. To overdose, you would have to take over 850 mcg. The overdose symptoms are hair loss, nail malformation, slow thinking, depression, and vomiting.

Silicon – is used by the body to strengthen connective tissue. If you get plenty of silicon with magnesium and calcium, your body will not allow aluminum to deposit and cause Alzheimer's disease. The brain uses a lot of silicon, and lack of it will affect your entire health.

Silicon is needed for good skin, nails, tendons, and hair health. Getting the right amount of silicon in your body will prevent falling hair. The silicon form that is found in your body tissues is silica. Silica in your hair strengths the hair and strengths the tissue at the hair root so that your hair does not pull out easily.

How do you know if you lack silica? Look at your fingernails. If you have lines or ridges on your nails, parallel to your fingers, then you are deficient in silica.

Zinc – deficiency has been linked to many-body conditions and illness. But, first you need to look at your fingernails. Do you have white spot in them? If you do, then, you mostly likely are deficient in zinc, and you need to take a good supplement.

If you work out you will lose zinc as you sweat. If use certain drugs, zinc will be used up by these drugs and eliminated in your urine.

Zinc is used by your entire reproductive system. Keeping an adequate supply of zinc in your blood can keep your prostate healthy and reduce body stress caused by an enlarged prostate. In her book, "The Food Pharmacy", 1988, Jean Carper says,

"And what happens to males who don't eat enough zinc? They don't mature sexually; their gonads shrink up. Also, normal males with zinc deficiencies fail to produce enough male hormone testosterone and sperm and can become infertile or impotent."

If you lack zinc, then you could exhibit these conditions:

- Rough hands
- Poor appetite – not eating that right foods does not provide the nutrients you need for your hair
- Delayed healing of wounds
- Reduced collagen
- Reduced body growth
- Poor immune system – you need a strong immune system to have healthy hair
- Acne – in acne follicles are plugging up and in thinning or loss of hair, your hair follicles are plugging up
- Weaken connective tissue.

If you are taking Amiloride, a diuretic drug to remove sodium from your body to lessen edema or hypertension, then you need to watch your zinc intake, since this drug will cause you to accumulate zinc. This problem is not seen, if you are taking the drug Triamterene. The side effects for too much zinc in your body are:

- Vomiting
- Stomach problems
- Metal taste in the mouth

Zinc foods — ginger root, organic or free range beef, liver, organic eggs, whole wheat, pecans, split peas, rye, oats, almonds, walnuts, lima beans, buckwheat, free-range chicken.

Oysters are the highest in zinc content than any other food.

Royal Jelly

There is a product called IRENA which is made in the UK by Irene Stein. This supplement contains royal jelly and the following nutrients:

Echinacea*
Gingko Biloba
Goldenseal
Horsetail
Rosemary
Saw Palmetto*
Yarrow
Calcium*

Magnesium*
Manganese*
Omega-3 Fatty Acid
Omega-6 Fatty Acid
Selenium
Vitamin A (Retinol)*
Vitamin B1 (Thiamin)*
Vitamin B12 (Cobalt)*
Vitamin B2 (Riboflavin)*
Vitamin B5 (Pantothenic Acid)*
Vitamin B6 (Pyridoxine)*
Vitamin B9 (Folic Acid)*
Vitamin C (Ascorbic Acid)*
Vitamin E*
Vitamin H (Biotin)*
Zinc*

Minerals

Minerals provide many functions in the body. They provide the charged ions that provide a battery across each body cell that allows movement of material in and out of your cells. They help build digestive and systemic enzymes and hormones. They form parts of blood, bone, cells, and body fluids, and hair.

The best way to get minerals into your body is to eat organic fruits and vegetables. Here are two ways that I recommend you supplement to get these nutrients.

I recently started using a product called '**Ruby Reds**." This product contains over 30 different fruit powders and many other nutrients. This combination provides you with a variety of balanced minerals and nutrients. Ruby Reds provide you with a high level of antioxidants and phytonutrients.

I also recommend you use a product called Trace-Lyte. This product contains minerals as crystalloids. Minerals in this form bypass the digestive process and are quickly absorbed.

Collagen

One super supplement to take to strengthen your hair is called **Super Collagen** + C so take this supplement with Hyaluronic Acid. Both these nutrients provide collagen for your skin, hair, joints, and many other body areas.

Aloe Vera

Aloe vera is an amazing herb. It has a list of healing powers you would not believe. But, for sure, it is capable of penetrating the skin to increase blood flow, reduce inflammation, kill bacteria, and heal the surface.

Aloe vera has antibiotic, antiviral and antifungal properties. This makes it ideal to use on the scalp for any infections caused by bacteria, virus, or fungus. Since it can penetrate the 7 layers of the skin, it is effective in most skin disorders – acne, psoriasis, eczema, or skin rashes.

Because of its ability easily penetrate the skin, aloe vera can be used as a media for substance you want to penetrate the skin.

Aloe vera gel can be used on your hair to correct an oily condition. One of the issues with hair loss is an excess of oil, which tends to plug up the hair follicles, which destroys the growth hair. Dandruff is also a condition that will create hair loss. Dandruff will accumulate on the scalp, mix with scalp oil and dirt to plug up follicles.

Aloe vera gel is one treatment for dandruff and excess scalp oil. Since it is capable of penetrating the skin, it can also penetrate the hair giving it a shining appearance and bulk.

Melatonin

So, what does melatonin have to do with hair loss? In clinical studies with rats, melatonin was shown to extent their life expectancy by 15 to 30%. Those rats that took melatonin had better fur for a longer period of time than those rats that did not take melatonin. It is the pineal gland, in the brain, that secretes melatonin and it slowly decreases the amount it gives the body as the body ages. It appears that when the pineal gland slows its melatonin output, it is telling the body to age. And, as you age and various body systems and organs deteriorate, you start to lose more hair.

You can keep your hair for a longer time in your life when you take melatonin. But, not by just taking melatonin, you must take other supplements and eat the food that keeps your whole body healthy and strong.

Most people I have worked with take 1-5 mg of melatonin. Some people have experience headaches when they take melatonin. Since melatonin is a hormone, it may have upset the balance of their hormones. If you get headaches, just don't use it. Perhaps one reason melatonin works so good is that it works in conjunction with the thymus gland, the master immunity gland, to helps protection you from illness and disease.

8: Eating for Hair Growth

Many people say they tried everything to grow hair, including changing their diet and taking supplements and nothing seems to works. In a survey that I did one respondent said,

"For the last year I have experienced patchy hair loss and thinning on the top front of my hair. I am very much into juicing, green foods, and blending. I have tried natural clay shampoos, essential oils, supplements and essential fatty acids. I used to have a beautiful crown of glory. I want my hair back, what can me do.? My research has been extensive but to no avail. I don't want to use Propecia or Rogaine. Please give me some information."

Another respondent said,

"Is it possible to totally regrow all of your lost hair permanently? I have tried all kinds of pills, potions and scalp exercises and nothing works....help????"

And here is the question that will be answered in this chapter,

"What must I eat to have a healthy hair?"

If you want to stop hair loss and grow your hair back, you need to concentrate on those foods that will help you regain your health. Most of us eat a diet of processed foods and foods that have very little nutritional value - nutrients, minerals, and vitamins. The results are that the body is starving for vitamins, minerals, enzymes, phytosterols, phytonutrients, bioflavonoids, and many other nutrients.

One of the first principles of eating to create good health and a full head of hair is:

Minimize the use of foods that make you thirsty. The body needs water, and that water needs to come from the foods you eat.

So let's get started.

You don't want to change your diet too fast. Each week change something that is bad for you and add something that is good. As you change your diet, there will be times when you eat food that is good for you, and you feel sick or have a stomach upset. This will pass as you continue to use this food. Your stomach has to get used to processing this new food. In addition, good food tends to cause the release of toxic matter in your body and it is these toxins that will make you feel sick.

Remember to take digestive enzymes with each meal.

Protein

You need plenty of protein to build cells, tissue, and hair, but not an excess. Proteins are the building block of your body and are active in hemoglobin, plasma, antibodies, hormones, and enzymes.

You need to absorb plenty of protein to grow hair and to stop it from falling out.

Meat should be the type that does not have coloring or preservatives. The animals should not have been contaminated with hormones or antibiotics. Normally you would buy this type of meat at a health food store like Whole Foods in the USA. Protein powers can be used but in limited amounts.

Most of you eat plenty of protein. Probably more than you need. But, of the all of the protein you eat, you don't absorb more than 20% of it. Simply because your body doesn't need much protein and you may not have enough minerals and vitamins to help digest and absorb the protein you eat. Without enough minerals in your body, you will not properly metabolize the protein that has gotten into your body.

Lack of protein just like excess protein causes your hair to go into the telogen cycle, resting cycle.

So what happens to the protein that is not used up? It becomes acidic, creating gout and needs minerals to neutralize it so it won't harm your tissue. The result is you lose more minerals and now you have even less for your hair growth or health. Can you see that if you don't eat or take plenty of minerals, you don't have a chance to even keeping the hair that you have and much less grow any.

So what happens to the protein that does not get absorbed? It bypasses the small intestines and goes into the colon. There in the colon, if you have not eaten enough fiber and other laxative promoting foods, you will get constipation. Constipation causes toxins that get back into the blood and then requires the help of minerals and anti-oxidants to neutralize them. And the worst part is that you are setting yourself up for various colon diseases, including colon cancer.

You need about 16 – 19% of protein calories in your diet. The amount of protein your body needs is about 25 – 60 grams, depending on your weight. Those of you that do physical work will need more for energy and strength.

For protein, eat clean meat, chicken, and fish. Do not eat pork because of the toxins and because the body has a hard time using this with this kind of protein. You can use soy products but you need to eat plenty of vegetable with soy, since soy uses up minerals during its digestion. Because most soy is now GMO it is problem best to go with milk or goat whey. Women and children should stay away from soy, since its main nutrient mimics estrogen.

In her book, Hair thru Diet, 1961, Katie Pugh points to a study where,

"Scientist doing research work with rats seems to be able to denude the rats at will by feeding them an average American diet but withholding such B-vitamins as inositol and choline as found in Brewer's Yeast and liver. Then growing hair back on the rats in a short time by giving them a wholesome diet plus the B-vitamins ..."

In the previous chapter, I listed the major nutrients that your hair needs to be healthy. In some of the foods listed here, you will be getting these nutrients. Always eat until you are satisfied but don't over eat. When you overeat you stress and overwork the body organs and overtime this weakens them.

For balanced eating, you need to eat the basic nutrient building blocks – protein, carbohydrates, and fats – but they must be quality foods.

Carbohydrates – Natural grains should be eaten and processed gain products like white bread, donuts, cakes, noodles, white rice, cookies, morning cereals should be limited.

Fats – Limit your fat intake to good fats. Minimize eating saturated fats like butter, bacon, cheese, milk. Eat less meat –beef or chicken - since they have high saturated fat content. Use olive oil and flax seed oil in your salads. You should supplement with fish-oil capsules daily.

Eat more foods with monounsaturated oil such as avocados, olive oil, almonds, cashews, pecans, pine nuts, pistachios, sunflower, seeds, pumpkin seeds, sesame seeds, rice bran, wheat bran, and oat bran.

Fiber - Fiber is critical for your health. Many people don't eat fruits and/or vegetables. This is a big mistake because this is the only way you can get the fiber, vitamins, minerals and nutrients that your body needs.

Lack of fiber affects digestion and assimilation of nutrients. It also is necessary for eliminating toxins and excess nutrients that your body does not need. When you don't eat enough fiber, food stays longer in the intestinal tract causing toxins and bacteria to form. These toxins can be absorbed into your blood, affecting the quality of your blood and function of cells.

Lack of fiber in your diet affects hair growth, because the quality of nutrients in your blood decreases.

Your main source of fiber should be from fruits, vegetables, and nuts or seeds. You can get fiber from grains but when cooked, they have no enzymes.

- Raw wheat germ
- brewer's yeast or nutritional yeast
- lecithin
- carrot juice
- vegetable oils
- honey
- kelp

- sunflower seeds or meal
- nuts
- all sorts of raw fruits that are grown in your location
- all sorts of raw vegetables that are grown in your location

Digestive enzymes

Your blood needs good nutrition and it gets it when you properly digest your food and absorb it through your small and large intestine. By the time you are 30 years, your digestive abilities has decreased considerably. To improve your digestion you need to take digestive enzymes at the start or after each meal.

Use a broadband digestive enzyme that contains amylase, protease, and lipase. If you are over 60 start testing to see if you need Betaine, HCL. The amount and strength of your stomach acid, HCL, decreases as you age and your ability to digest proteins and fats decreases. Without a good amount of HCL which has a pH of 1.5 to 2.1, you cannot properly process protein and process calcium, B12, and iron. Even more important is the lack of HCL limits the destruction of bad bacteria and micro-organisms - Salmonella, E.coli, and C. difficile.

Probiotics

Probiotics refers to live good bacteria that you have in your stomach, intestines, and colon. It is live bacteria that you should supplement your diet with. You have over 500 species of good and bad bacteria spread throughout your gastrointestinal tract, starting in your mouth and ending in your anus. These bacteria are at constantly at war with each other, each trying to dominate. The most important thing about bacteria is that you must have more good bacteria than bad, so that the good bacteria can maintain control of your gastrointestinal tract and provide you with the health benefit of having good bacteria.

If you have history of using antibiotics or have recently used them, then you need to use a good probiotics for a least a month. Using antibiotics kills both good and bad bacteria. This allows bad bacteria to take over your gastrointestinal tract and produce toxins and excretions that are bad, for your blood and body functions.

Once bad bacteria take over it is hard to re-establish your good bacteria, but using a good probiotics can help you do this. Using probiotics helps your digestion and makes your intestinal tract more alkaline, making it difficult for bad bacteria to thrive.

Good bacterial also helps you create vitamin K, B12, and Biotin.

Here is a list of good bacteria that you can find in supplements, where the L stands for Lactobacillus.

- L. Acidophilus
- L. Bifidus
- L. Bulgaricus

- S. Thermophilus
- L. Casei

The most common good bacteria are the first three in this list. When you buy probiotics, only buy a supplement with a few strains of good bacteria, since they compete with each other to take over the intestinal area.

Special Morning Smoothie

Here is a morning smoothie that will help you stop hair loss, promote hair growth, and help you get your day started right. This smoothie will provide you with various nutrients and protein needed for hair health. You can vary the ingredients and vary the proportions until you create something you really like. Try to use organic products when possible.

In a blender, put the following ingredients,

- One banana
- Fresh or frozen strawberries or any other type of fruit
- I cup or more of apple juice or any other type of fruit juice
- One scoop of Super Red powder
- One tablespoon or more of flaxseed oil
- One tablespoon of nutritional yeast

- One tablespoon of lecithin granules

- One ½ scoop of protein whey

- One tablespoon of wheat germ

- One or two tablespoons of your favorite liquid probiotics.

Now blend for 1 -2 minutes or until everything is blended properly. Drink this every morning when possible. You can add small amounts of other liquids or nutrients, like rice dream or almond milk. When you drink this smoothie you can take a capsule of B-vitamins and 2000mg of MSM.

Foods and Habits to Avoid

You should avoid most processed foods. These foods are not only deficient in nutrients but pull vitamins and minerals out of your body to process them. If you eat a lot of processed food, you will mostly likely not be able to gain good hair health. It will not matter how many supplements you take.

Sugar

Sugar is a prime cause of loss of hair. Not only does it cause hair loss, but, it is responsible for stimulating and starting many other diseases. It is so detrimental to your health that it is amazing that it has not been outlawed. If you are able to eliminate this addictive substance from your diet, you will see a marked improvement in your health and in the health of your hair.

When sugar cane is processed to create sugar, 90% or more of the original minerals in sugar cane are lost – magnesium, chromium cobalt, copper, zinc, and manganese. When you eat sugar, you pull minerals and vitamins out of your body to help digest and process this sugar. Any time you use up minerals to do something other than build your body, your body becomes more acid and susceptible disease and loss of hair.

Smoking

If you smoke, you are wasting your time trying to grow hair or stop hair loss. However, if you have genes for thick hair, even smoking will not stop your hair growth. If you took the nutrients recommended here most of them would go to offset the intake of the free radicals and toxins created by smoking.

Nicotine will reduce the amount of blood that flows to your scalp by constricting the veins and reducing the pumping action of your heart. In addition, the carbon monoxide that is created by smoking interferes with the use of oxygen in the cells and throughout the body. Oxygen is one element that is needed metabolize or burn the various nutrients to feed your hair.

Salt

If you need to use salt in your food, change to sea salt.

Sea salt is a natural balance of various minerals and creates less damage in your body than regular salt. But it is always best to avoid all salt, since many foods you eat have salt and you don't even know it. Excess use of salt increases the amount of water that your body stores. This causes an increase in blood pressure and excess water, lymph liquid, around your cells that can lead to edema.

Sodium is a mineral that helps maintain a voltage charge, a battery, across your cell walls in partnership with potassium. Sodium is more plentiful outside your cells than it is inside your cells. And, there is more potassium inside your cells than outside. Since these minerals exist in an electrical form, they create a battery across the cell, which causes minerals and nutrients to enter your cells. This battery also helps to pull out used minerals and nutrients or waste out of your cells. This is the nature of good health and this process should not be disturbed.

When you eat table salt, sodium, which your body does not need, this sodium ends up in the lymph liquid around your cells. This excess sodium attracts water, which floods the area around your cells. When this happens, you will have decreased battery energy across the cell membrane. Now your health is compromised and the health of your hair is diminished.

Clinical studies have shown that bald men have higher blood pressure than non-bald men. As we have seen in many studies that diet and an excess of salt leads too high blood pressure. In some countries that use only natural flavoring in food, no salt, men do not become bald.

Here are more foods to avoid:

White Flour Packaged foods, canned fruits, cold cereals, soft drinks, pork caffeinated coffee, candy, alcohol

9: Reduce Stress for Hair Growth

Just seeing your hair thinning or becoming bald can cause you stress that adds another problem to those you might already have. This in turn increases your stress and can cause you to lose more hair.

If you haven't hear this, "You can be doing every healthy thing for your body, but if you have high stress, you will still be unhealthy", now you have.

When you are under stress or receive shocking news, you release adrenaline and cortisol. Adrenaline decreases digestion and slows down colon movement. Whereas, cortisol destroys brain cells and reduces your immune system.

You also stress your body when you don't get enough sleep or when you work on swing or grave shifts. These shifts go against your natural living cycle. Also, you stress your body when you don't get enough sunlight. Working and living under artificial light stresses your body and shortens your life span. Florescent light is the most harmful light, because of the 60 cycle flickering that is picked up by your brain causing your body stress.

There is lighting that you can buy that gives off a full spectrum of light frequencies that emulate natural light.

Watch your stress level. Learn how to relax more by using hypnosis or hemi-sync CD's. If you use antacids for **acid reflux or heartburn**, stop using them since they reduce your ability to absorb vitamins, and this adds stress to your body. Start using digestive enzymes each time you eat. Digestive enzymes are good for everyone. You save your own internal digestive enzymes, when you use a supplement.

Adrenals

If you are experiencing adrenal exhaustion from excess stress, then here are some of the symptoms you might have are:

- Low blood sugar levels
- Tiredness
- Allergies
- Muscle weakness
- Thinning hair
- Grooved fingernails
- Low body temperature–this is also a symptom of hypothyroidism
- Constipation

Stress has a large factor in how healthy your hair is, since it creates malnutrition. Stress results in loss of various nutrients that are necessary for good health and hair stability and growth.

10: Exercise That Helps Grow Hair

Caution: If you have not exercised for a while, take this program slowly and work into it. If you feel some concern about exercising and your health, make sure you see your doctor before exercising.

As I have mentioned, you need a good cardiovascular system to support great hair. The slow degradation of your cardiovascular system is reflected in your hair as hair loss, hair thinning, and balding. Of course, there could be other causes of your hair loss, but 80% of the time this will be the cause. Also, if you add other causes such as using drugs, poor diet or stress to a slowly deteriorating cardiovascular system, you will get the other 20%.

So let's get started with the exercises you need to do. You will be doing these exercises in a different way than you are used to. Most exercise gurus tell you that you need aerobics to strengthen your hearts. Exercise studies have shown that this is not the way to strengthen your heart; in fact, it does the opposite. When you go to the gym to do repetitive exercises for over 20 minutes, you are not strengthening your heart or going to lose weight that will stay off.

In his e-book called **Pace**, Dr. Al Sears, outlines a

new way of exercising to strengthen your cardiovascular system. He says that,

"During twenty years of working with extremely fit athletes, patients with diseased or injured hearts, and average people in between, one thing is apparent. Doing what we have come to accept as 'cardio' exercise is a waste of your time and effort.

It doesn't build what your heart really needs. It doesn't increase your heart's ability to respond to the real demands. In fact, for all your effort, you only reduce your ability to handle suddenly demanding events that may come your way – the last thing you want."

During the short, fast exercises from 2 to 15 minutes, you are burning calories supplied by:

- The first couple of minutes the energy comes from your ATP – cell energy.

- After 2 minutes the energy comes from the carbohydrates stored in your muscle tissue

- After 15-20 minutes the energy starts to come from stored fat
- When you exercise is at a moderate rate, you are burning 40% carbohydrates and 55% fat. When you exercise at a high intensity, you are burning 95% carbohydrates and 3% fat.

You want to exercise in a way and time duration where you are burning carbohydrates and very little fat.

When you exercise and burn fat, you are telling your body that you need fat when you exercise. So when you come to exercise next time, your body will have stored fat to sustain the energy you need during exercising. Your body is storing and building up your fat reservoirs each time you eat so it can sustain the moderate-intensity exercises that you do.

So, you want to do fast short exercising and not moderate long exercising.

One other thing, when you are just at your rest state, not exercising, you are burning 35% carbohydrates and 65% fat. What this means is that you will continue to store fat if you do not exercise at all. You are telling your body that when you do nothing, you need fat to be able to do nothing. So when you eat, your body will store fat from the food you eat. No exercise is a destructive activity for your body.

If you practice high-intensity exercise, chances of a heart disease are 100% less than those who do aerobic exercise.

Now as far as hair health, having a good cardiovascular system will increase your chances of limiting, minimizing, or even stopping hair loss.

Anaerobic Exercise

The way you will exercise is to exercise for a short duration at high intensity. This is called anaerobic exercise. To do anaerobic exercise, you exercise at a pace you can't sustain for more than a short time. You will be breathing hard and are asking your lungs for more oxygen than they can give you.

Because of this your lungs need to expand to get more oxygen. You are now building your lungs for greater capacity. You are now burning more carbohydrates than fat. And, in the time between exercising your fat is burned, since your body determines it is not necessary to keep fat for energy since carbohydrates are what is really needed.

So what are the benefits for your hair, by doing anaerobic exercise?

- Reverse heart disease
- Lower cholesterol
- Reduce high blood pressure
- Increase oxygen contain in your blood
- Increase lung capacity
- Strengthen your immune system
- Reverse changes of aging

All of these benefits create cleaner arteries and more blood flow to your hair bringing more oxygen and more nutrients to your roots.

Exercising

As you do Pace exercising, you will change your routine each time you exercise. Instead of exercising longer, you will increase the exercise intensity and the resistive element of exercising.

To start this exercise program, start with a 10 minute workout. You can do your exercise on a stair-stepper, stationary bike, treadmill, and by running, swimming, or riding your bike. You will want to check with your doctor, if you:

- Have not a medical checkup during the past two years
- Are over 50
- Are 26 lbs. overweight
- Have heart pains, chest pains, or rapid heart palpitations after you exercise
- Are taking heart medication or have a pace maker
- Have angina, heart murmur or any type of heart disease
- Have a relative that died of a heart attack before the age of 60
- Have hard time breathing and have any type of respiratory disease – asthma, emphysema, or TB

Monitoring Your Heart Rate

To check your progress in your exercise program, you need to check your:
- Resting heart rate

- Maximum heart rate for your age
- Maximum heart rate during exercise
- Recovery heart rate

Resting Heart Rate

Your resting heart rate is before you exercise. The lower your resting heart rate is the healthier you are, unless you have a pacemaker or heart problems. Normal rate is 60 to 100 pulses per minute. If you are really in good shape, then your pulse may be 40 – 60 per minute

To determine your resting heart rate, get a second timer and count the number of pulses you have in 10 seconds. Then, multiple this number by 6, to get your pulse rate per minute. To get a more accurate reading of your pulse rate, do you 10 second reading 3 times and get an average of these readings.

Maximum Heart Rate for Your Age

The maximum heart rate for your age is that heart rate that you should strive for during your exercise, to get the best benefit of your exercise. You calculate this rate by subtracting your age from 220. During your exercise, you want to achieve 60- 80 % of your maximum heart rate for your age. Here is a sample chart you can use to see different heart rates for your heart:

Age	Max Pulse 220-age	60% of max pulse	80% of max pulse
35	185	111	148
40	180	108	144
45	175	105	140
50	170	102	136
55	165	99	132
60	160	96	128
65	155	93	124
70	150	90	120

Based on your physical condition, use these numbers as guide lines.

Maximum Heart Rate During Exercise

The maximum heart rate is the highest rate your pulse achieved during your exercise. Use the chart above to evaluate where you are with respect to the heart rate for your age. During exercise if your heart rate is on the lower end of the heart rate for your age, you will want to exercise harder to get your heart rate up. If you are really out of shape, then take it easy and work up to the 60% and eventually to the 80% heart rate, as you improve your stamina.

You can measure your exercise heart rate the same way you calculate your resting heart rate.

Recovery Heart Rate

The heart recovery rate is the time it takes for your maximum heart rate to recover to your resting heart rate. As you exercise more, the less time will be required for you to achieve your heart recovery rate. When you exercise for your chosen time, clock your recovery rate, since a change in this rate indicates you are improving in your healthy. You will see change in this rate in one month.

Do not do your next exercise until you reach your resting heart rate. So you will be cycling from resting rate –exercise rate – resting rate – exercise rate – resting rate. Do ten of these cycles as on exercise routine.

Caution: See your doctor before you start an exercise program or if the following conditions occur:

- Your heart rate, after maximum exercise, does not come
- down within a few minutes
- You feel dizzy or faint
- You have chest pains or are short of breath
- You have rapid heartbeat or irregular heartbeat

This exercise program is the basic outline of Dr. Sears' **PACE program**. His e-book takes off to higher levels of exercise methods, so if you want to see his full program you can buy his e-book called Pace.

11: About The Author And Other Resources

Get one of my best kindle books *free* below:

http://www.natural-remedies-thatwork.com

Rudy Silva is a natural nutritional consultant educated in the United States in Nutrition and Physics. He is a graduate from San Jose State University in California. He is author of 45 other books on natural remedies. He has authored a newsletter in natural remedies for over 10 years.

Resource page

Here are some of the other kindle e-books about natural remedies that have been written by this author. You can see the entire list at:

http://tinyurl.com/b2f7wd3

Acne Remedies

- Best natural acne treatments: Acne facial
- Effective Acne Treatments That Work

Constipation Remedies

- The Best Constipation Remedies

- Best Constipated Women Natural Cures
- How To Relieve Constipation With Fruits

Essential Fatty Acids

- Taking The Mystery Out Of Essential Fatty acids
- Amazing Fish Oil Benefits Revealed
- Omega 3 and 6 Mystery Exposed

Nutrition Remedies

- Updated Version - Secret Diet And Nutrition
- Secret Healthy Fruit Practices Revealed
- Fast Healing Juice Nutrition Therapy: Nutrition Tips 3
- Fantastic Alkaline Fruit Benefits Revealed
- Calcium (Discover How To Use Calcium To Avoid Devastating Diseases)
- Magnesium Nutrition Revealed
- Best Nutrition Health Practices
- Potassium Health Secrets Revealed
- Phosphorus, The Best Brain Food
- A Sodium Diet (What You Must Know About Sodium)
- Vegetables and Vegetable Juice Cures
- Alkaline Body: How to Change an Acid Body into an Alkaline body

Stomach Remedies

- Acid Reflux: Fast and Easy Cures For Acid Reflux
- Asthma Treatment Cures With Remedies
- How To Do Natural Colon Cleansing
- Gastrointestinal Digestion Secrets Revealed

Misc Remedies

- Natural Hair Loss Treatment: Women And Men
- Effective Natural Hemorrhoids Treatment
- Iron Deficiency Anemia
- Secrets To Understanding Behavior
- Fast Acting Ear Infection Remedies
- Best Behavior Secrets Revealed That Can Change Your Personality
- What Is A Hiatus Hernia
- Best Varicose Vein Treatments?
- Make Shampoos At Home Using Natural Ingredients:Discover recipes for quality natural hair shampoos
- How To Fix Your Thyroid Problems: Discover Hidden Ideas That Fix Your Thyroid

Minerals

- Calcium and Magnesium Magic Body Benefits Revealed
- The Magic of Sodium, Calcium and Magnesium
- Create an Alkaline Body with Potassium and Sodium: Eliminate a Potassium Deficiency

- Calcium and Phosphorus Foods: Deficiency or Excesses in These Minerals Cause Bone and Brain Power Loss
- Chlorine The Body Detoxifier (With water, chlorine will clean your body of toxins and pathogens)

Men's Health

- Best Impotence Health Diet

Weight loss

- Ten (10) Day Quick Success Weight Loss Program: A new approach to losing weight by changing your eating habits for life
- Discover Secret Anti-Aging Juice & Tonic Recipes: Unique Juices And Tonics That Create Beauty And Youth

To see all the kindle books written by this author, go to this the Authors Profile Page or this URL: http://tinyurl.com/b2f7wd3

If you need support or want to promote any of his e-books, please contact him at rss41@yahoo.com and expect a reply within 24 hours. He looks forward to hearing from you and is happy to help you understand his material on natural and nutritional health.

Give A Review

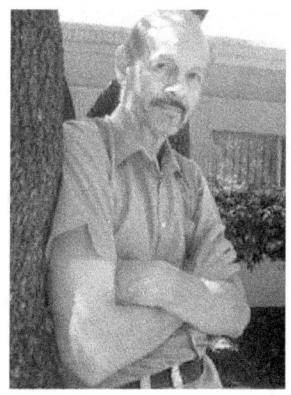

And, don't for get to give a review for this e-book at Amazon so that others can gain the benefits of what is in this e-book. To you, for losing weight, creating better health and more happiness in your life,

Rudy S Silva

www.ingramcontent.com/pod-product-compliance
Lightning Source LLC
Chambersburg PA
CBHW070801290526
45795CB00002B/586